Gentle Yoga

for

50 Plus

By Subodh Gupta

Corporate Yoga Trainer

First Edition September 2007

Copyright @2007 by Subodh Gupta

ISBN 978-1-84799-149-2
Library of Congress Control Number: 2007908785

Published by
Subodh Gupta
Headquarter: London (UK)
Email: info@subodhgupta.com
Website: www.subodhgupta.com

Publisher Note:
The reader should not regard the recommendations and Gentle Yoga exercises expressed and described in this book as substitute advice of a qualified medical practitioner. It is also advisable that reader may learn the gentle yoga exercise initially in presence of a qualified yoga trainer.

Acknowledgements

I am grateful to my parents and all my teachers who taught me at various stages of my life & shared with me their wisdom.

Begin your gentle yoga exercise with your wonderful smile.

SMILE please

Content

Practice Gentle Yoga

Daily

Slowly

With Awareness

Introduction:

This book of gentle yoga is specifically for those people who feel their body is stiff or has never done yoga before and wants to start yoga practice in the safest possible way to achieve healthy body and mind.

Gentle yoga can be practiced by anybody whether young or old, beginner or advance.

In my opinion these are the most important exercises for progressing into higher stages of yoga system by loosening up body joints, relaxing muscles and prepare healthy body & mind for meditation purpose.

These exercises are also recommended if suffering from arthritis or rheumatism.

The knowledge and technique of gentle yoga exercises are explained in this book in a step by step method along with precautions so that everybody can easily understand.

In the end I would like to say practicing gentle Yoga should be pleasant and enjoyable. If you do it regularly, gently with breath awareness they would certainly bring good health to you over a period of time.

May all being be healthy.

Subodh Gupta

"Yoga means Union"

Part 1

Understanding about Yoga posture

Whenever we hear about yoga the first thought comes to the mind is some sort of acrobatic postures or some kind of posture or pose which seems to be impossible to perform.

The most important point in Yoga practice is not flexibility and ability to do acrobatic postures, but awareness of the body and breath. *I repeat awareness of the body and breath.*

No matter how physically difficult posture you are able to do but if it is without your focused attention and awareness of breath then it is practice of a beginner. However even if you are doing physically seemingly easy gentle yoga posture or exercise with complete awareness of body and breath then it is considered as an advance practice of yoga system.

What is gentle yoga and why it is important?

If you wake up early morning and happen to see a cat or a dog waking up, you would be amazed to observe that first thing they do in the morning is some gentle stretches which help their body to get them back in working order. These little animals seem to know important knowledge about stretches from their basic instinct.

Although at first glance these gentle stretches may seem something insignificant, however practically they are very important even though these gentle stretches may not look as impressive as some of the unnecessary glorifying yoga postures (*which do not serve any practical purpose to most of the people except injuring some*) described in certain famous yoga books.

You can notice many people in their 60's start having various joints pain, lower back pain, neck pain etc for various reasons. The reasons could be our bad sitting postures, unhealthy life style, lack of physical movement, etc.

Muscles which are not used regularly become weak over a period of time and joints become stiff and free flow of energy in the body is obstructed which later on in old age create various kind of pain in body at various locations.

Let's understand with the help of an example:

Water which is flowing freely in the river under the sunlight tends to remain fresh, however stagnant water in any pond tends to get stale and germinate mosquito, similarly if energy is flowing freely in our body, our body tends to remain healthy and if energy is obstructed for a long time, it create pain and disease.

Gentle yoga consists of series of gentle exercises for various body joints which are practiced with breath awareness. These exercises help in releasing any trapped energy by exercising in gentle, effective and safe way. These exercises also make our muscles relaxed, supple, strong and joints get loosen up.

Regular practice will certainly lead you towards healthy body and mind.

Notes for Gentle Yoga Practitioners

Breathing through nose or mouth: Always breathe through the nose with the awareness (unless specified by mouth). *Remember a simple concept that by nature, mouth is for eating and nose is for breathing.* Please do not try to reverse the nature functions. As you breathe in, know that you are breathing in. As you breathe out, know that you are breathing out. This will greatly enhance your general health and well-being.

Just for the enlightment, nose performs not only the breathing function but it filters the air, moisturise the air, warms the air, it can smell, it secretes the mucus and performs many more functions etc.

Now think for a moment if the mouth can perform all these functions…….........................

Yes you are thinking correctly, mouth cannot perform all these functions, so please do not breathe through mouth unless specified in some special exercises.

Place of practice: It is good to practice in a room which is well ventilated. Please do not practice under a fan or direct sunlight.

Posture for doing Gentle Yoga: Any comfortable sitting position is ok. The main point is body needs to be relaxed and back straight. Do not slump and do not lean forward. It is good to sit on folded blanket or cloth which is made from natural fibre.

In case if you find it difficult to sit on the floor in cross leg sitting position, some of the gentle yoga postures described in this book can also be practiced while sitting on chair or while lying down on floor.

Relaxation: Whenever you feel tired during the practice of gentle yoga exercise, please relax and lie down on floor on your back for 2 to 3 minutes and practice slow and deep abdominal breathing described in this book at the end.

Deer abdominal breathing should be practiced for about 5 minutes after completing the gentle yoga exercise.

Practice Time of Gentle yoga: Gentle yoga exercise can be practiced any time during the day except just after the meals. However the best time for practice is early morning during sunrise or around sunset.

Awareness during Gentle Yoga: It is very important that while practicing gentle yoga, you are aware of your breath and body movement.

Any yoga posture without awareness of breath is a practice of a beginner.

Frequency of Practice: In my view everybody should practice gentle yoga everyday for at least 20 to 30 minutes.

Cautions: If you are suffering from any kind of neck related pain, injury or have gone through any recent operation, please consult your doctor first before beginning any of gentle yoga exercises.

Always remember Golden Rule:

Never *strain yourself while practicing gentle yoga*

Part2

Gentle Yoga Exercises

Exercise 1

Neck: Forward and back bending

Preparation: Sit in a cross-legged pose with hands resting on your knees with back straight (*You can also sit on the chair with your back straight if you find sitting on the floor with cross leg position inconvenient to you*).

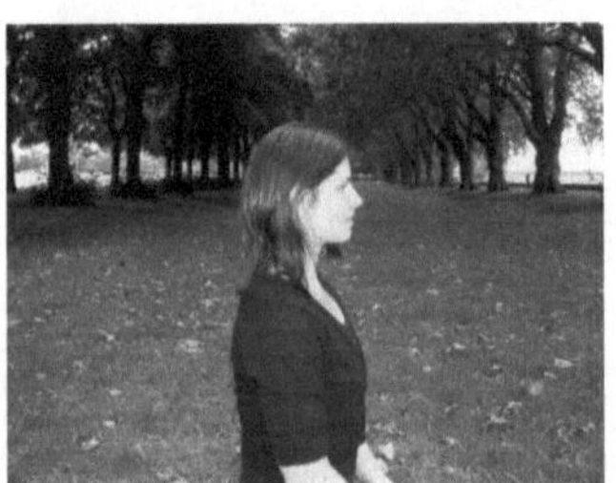

Caution: There should not be any strain in any neck movement. You can take your head forward and back only to the point where you feel absolutely comfortable.

Step1: As you exhale slowly bring your head down.

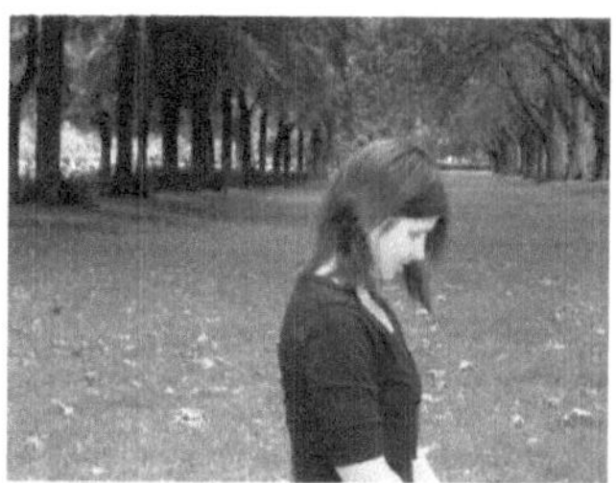

Step2: As you inhale move your head back as far as you feel comfortable.

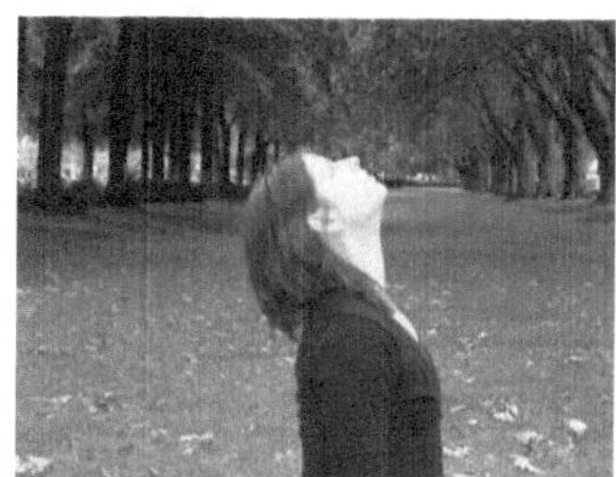

This is one round.

Practice 5 rounds.

Exercise2
Neck: Chin over shoulder

Preparation: Sit in a cross-legged pose with hands resting on your knees with back straight.

Step1: As you exhale turn your head towards your right shoulder.

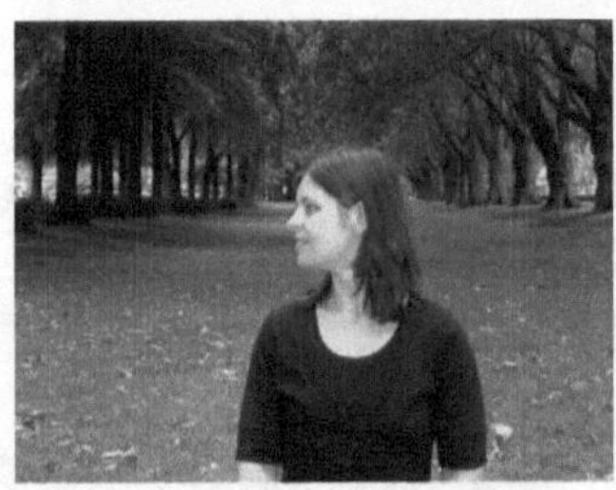

Step2: Inhale and bring the head to the centre position.

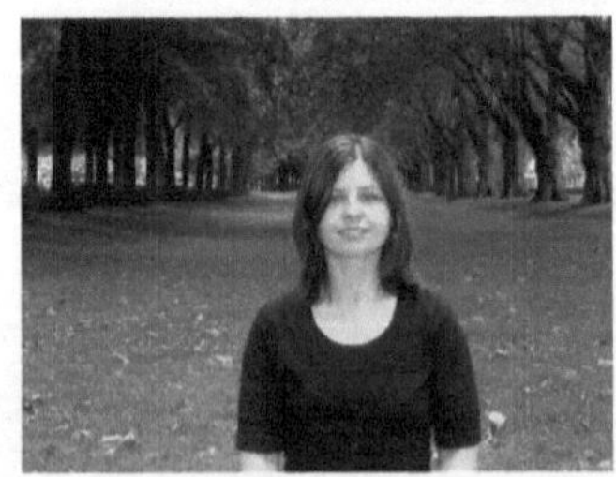

Step3: As you exhale turn your head towards your left shoulder.

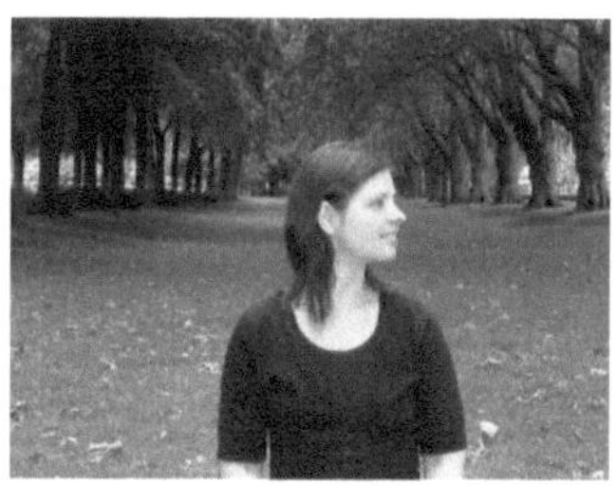

Step4: Inhale and bring the head to the centre.

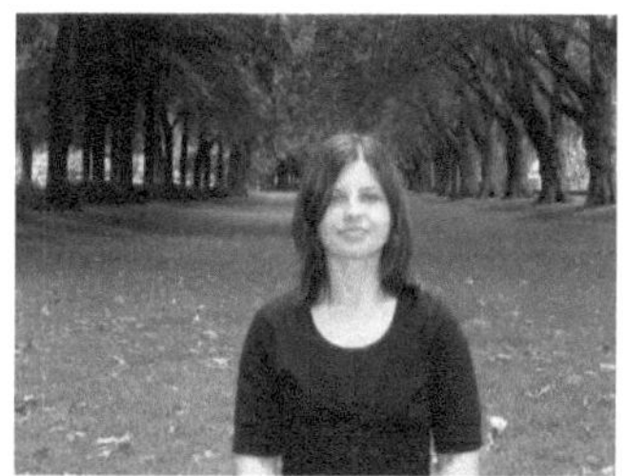

(This is one round)

Practice 5 rounds.

Exercise 3
Neck: Ear to shoulder movement

Preparation: Sit in a cross-legged pose with hands resting on your knees with back straight.

Step1: As you exhale lower your head toward your right shoulder (lowering right ear towards your right shoulder as shown in the picture).

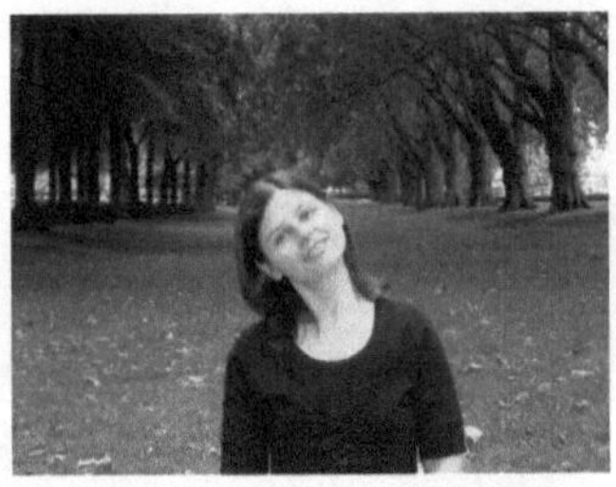

Step2: Inhale and come back to the centre.

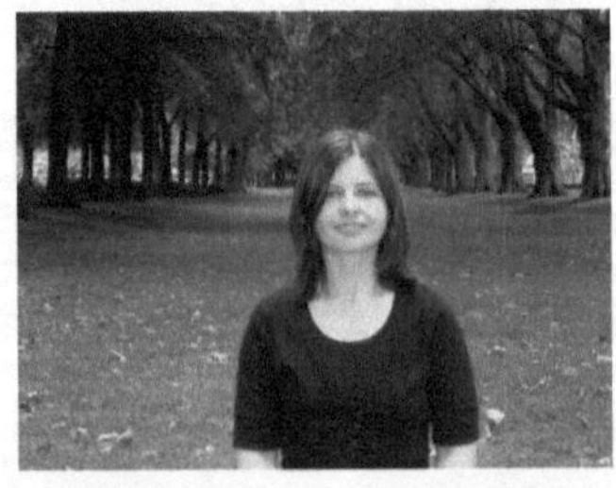

Step3: As you exhale lower your head toward your left shoulder.

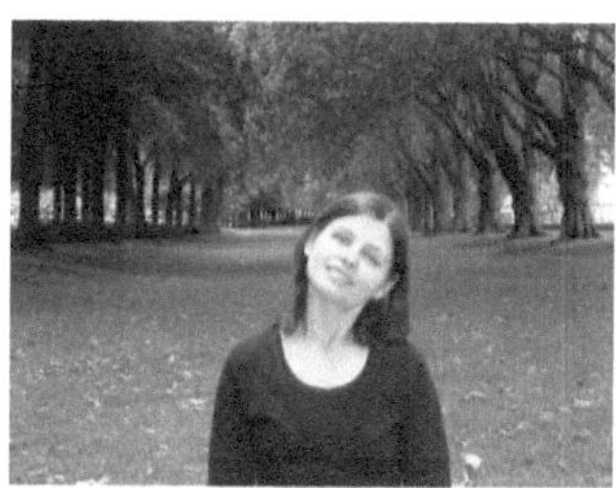

Step4: Inhale and come back to the centre (these all steps complete one round).

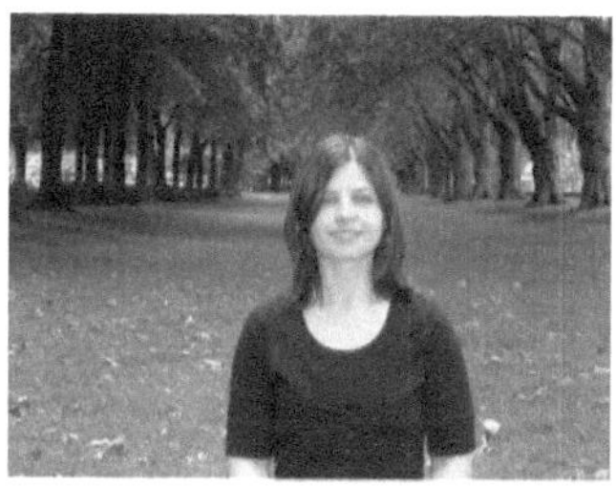

Practice 5 rounds.

Benefits:

These 3 neck exercises release tension and stiffness in the head, neck and shoulders, especially after prolonged work at the desk.

Precautions:

If you are suffering from any kind of neck related pain, injury or cervical spondylosis, please consult your doctor first before beginning any of gentle neck exercises.

Note: *The shoulders should not move in any of the neck exercises. Please be aware while practicing neck movement that only the neck and head should move.*

Exercise 4
Shoulder rotation

Preparation: Sit in a crossed-legged position with your back straight (*or you may sit on chair with your back straight if you find it difficult to sit on floor with cross leg position*).

Place your fingers on your shoulders with elbows down.

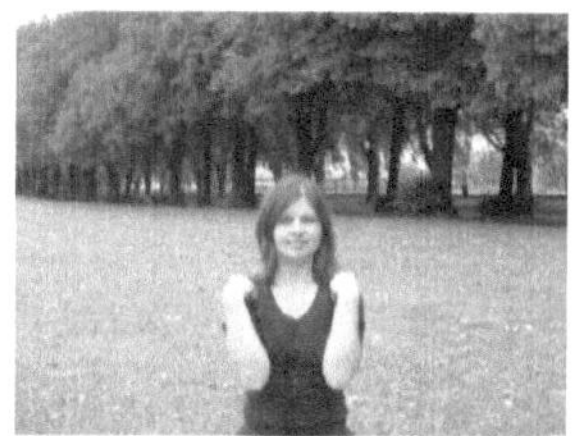

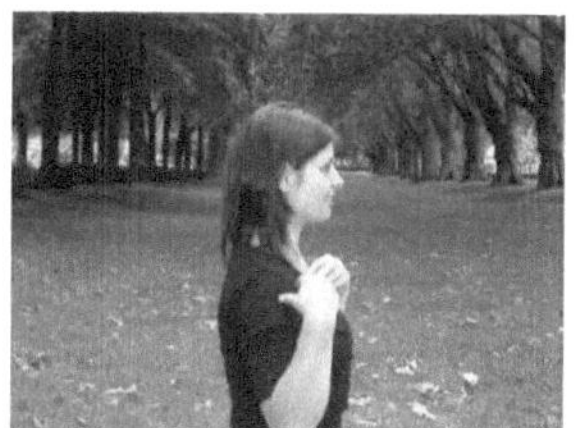

Step1: As you inhale rotate your shoulders upward (*elbows going up towards the ceiling as shown in the picture below*).

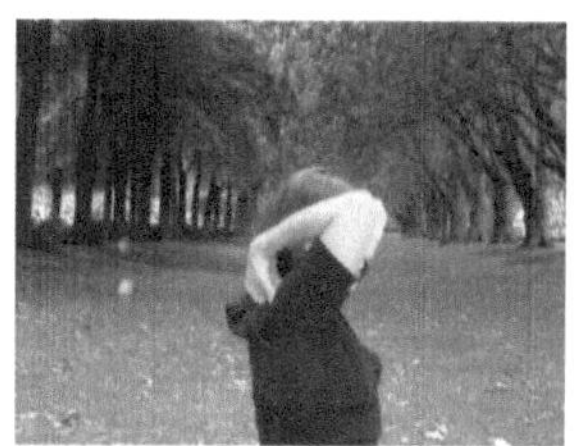

Step2: As you exhale fully rotate your shoulders downward (elbows going down towards the floor as shown in picture below).

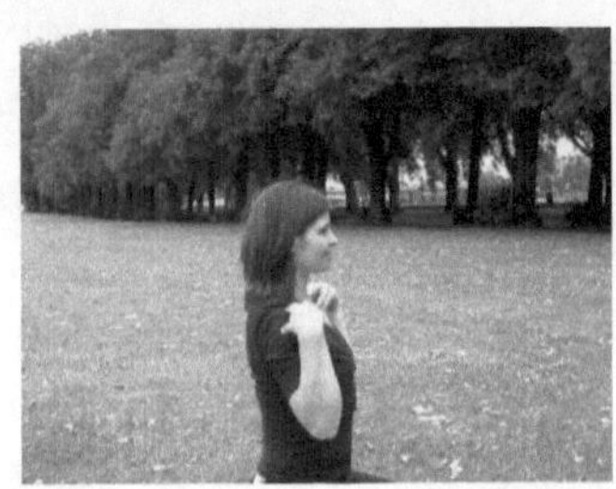

This completes one round.

Practice 5 rounds clockwise and 5 rounds anticlockwise.

Benefits:

This shoulder movement release the strain of driving, long hours of office work and also helpful in bringing mobility to tight shoulders.

Exercise 5
Elbow bending

Preparation: Stretch your arms in front of you, at shoulder level, palms facing up.

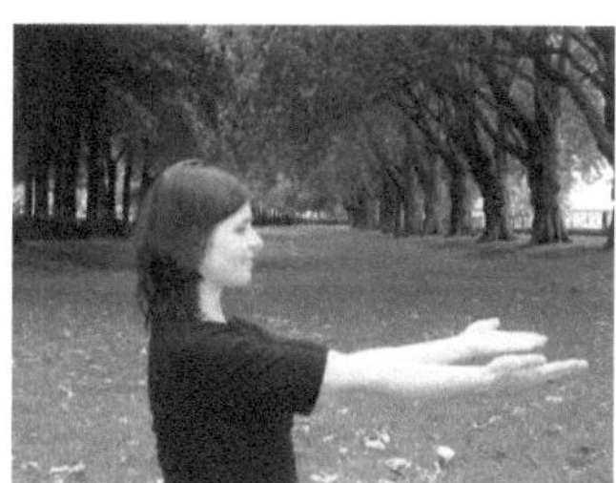

Step1: As you exhale, bend the arms at the elbow joints and bring the fingers to touch the shoulders, (as shown in picture).

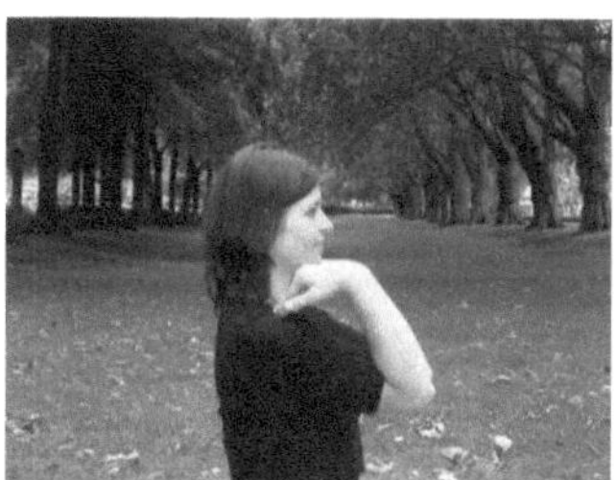

Step2. As you inhale stretch the arms.

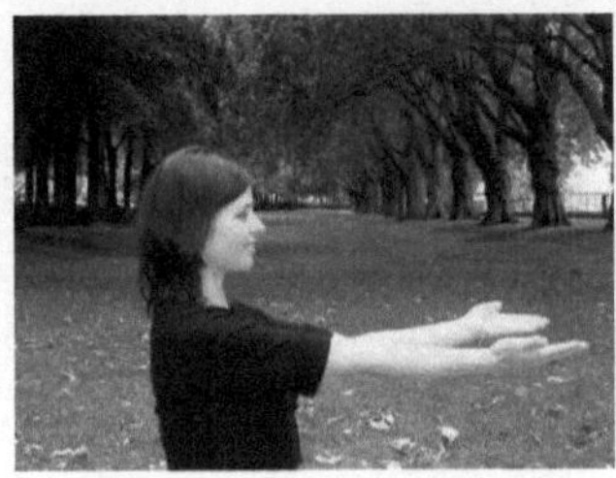

This completes one round.

Practice 5 rounds.

The following 3 gentle exercises are helpful in relieving tension in hands and wrists caused by prolong hours of working on computer or using your blackberry.

These movements are also beneficial in case of arthritis of the joints.

Exercise 6
Wrist bending

Preparation: Stretch your arms in front of you, at the shoulder level, palms facing down.

Step1. As you inhale bring your hands upward, so the fingers are pointing toward the ceiling, as shown in picture below.

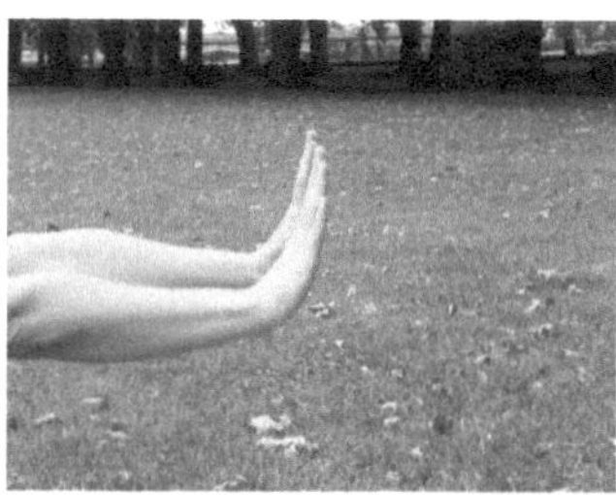
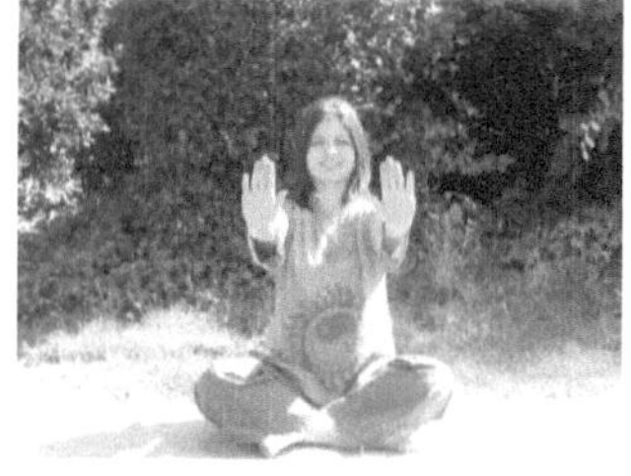

Step2. As you exhale bring your hands downward, so the fingers are pointing toward the floor, as shown in picture (this completes one round).

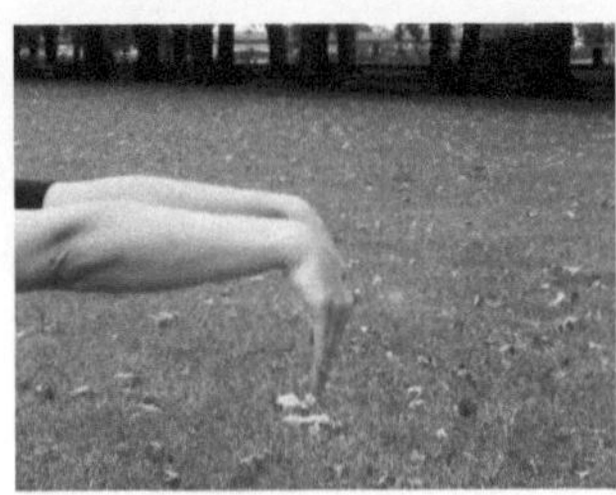 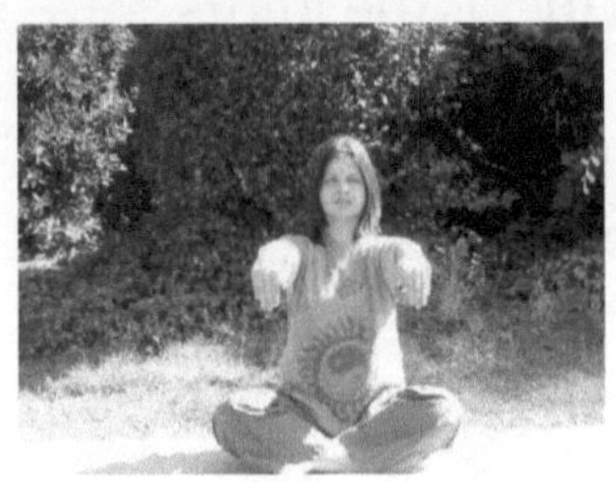

Practice 10 rounds.

Exercise7
Wrist joint rotation

Preparation: Stretch both your arms in front of you, at the shoulder level with the fists clenched.

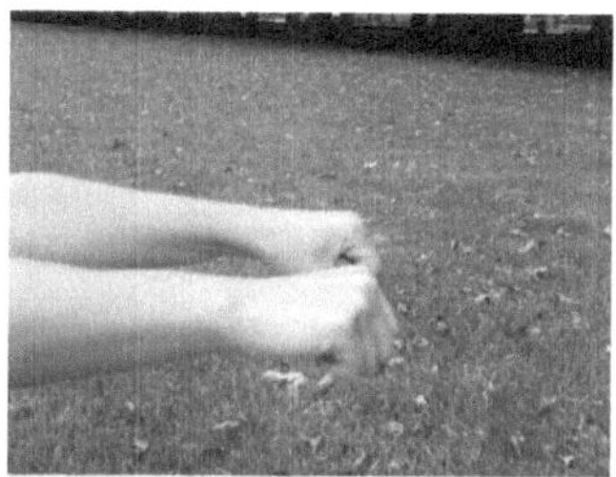

Step1. As you inhale rotate both of your fists upward, keeping the fists facing downward.

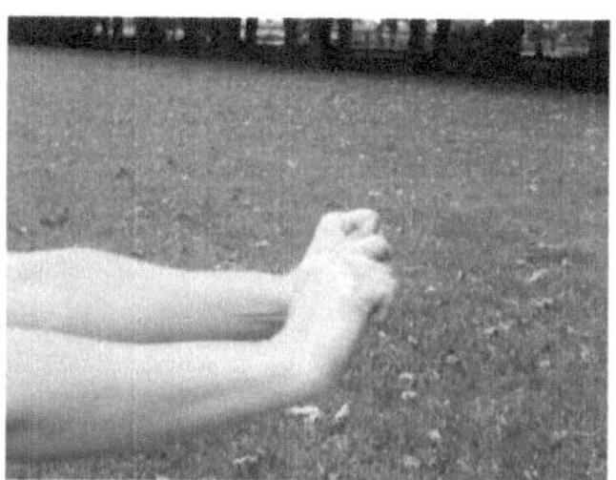

Step2. As you exhale rotate the fists downward.

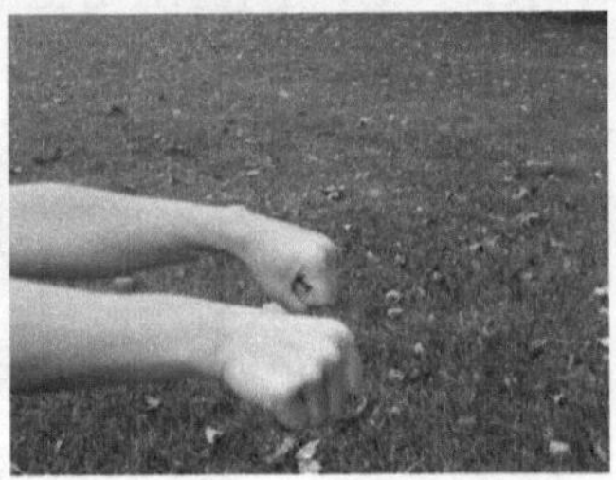

This completes one round.

Practice 5 rounds in each direction, clockwise and anticlockwise.

Exercise 8
Hand clenching

Preparation: Bring your arms straight in front of you, at the shoulder level.

Step1. As you inhale open your hands, keeping your palms down. Stretch your fingers as wide as you can.

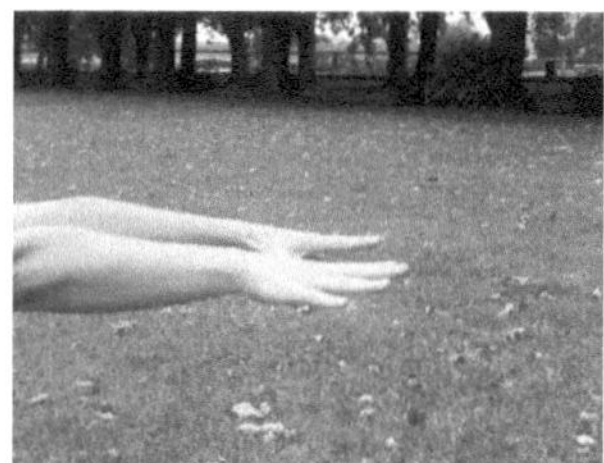

Step2. As you exhale make fists with your fingers.

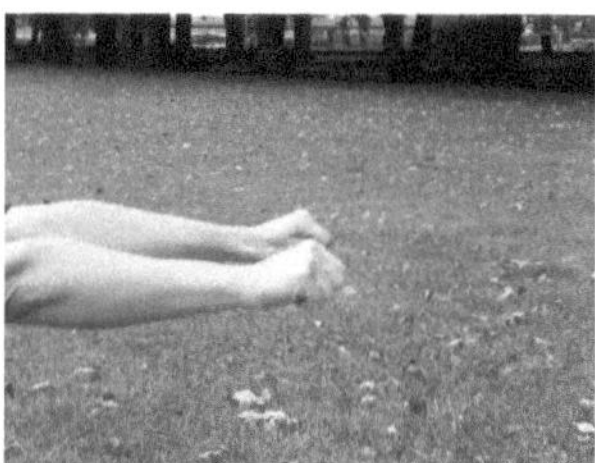

This completes one round.
Repeat 20 times.

Exercise 9
Hands in and out movement

Preparation: Stand straight or sit in a cross leg position with your arms in front of you at shoulder height and palms together as shown in the photo.

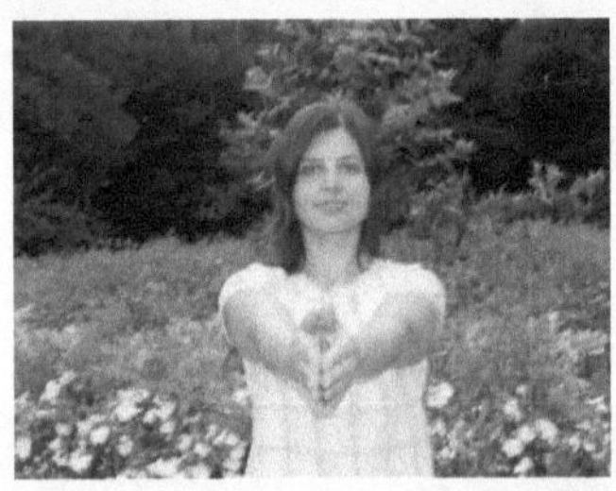

Step1: Now as you inhale, spread your arms slowly to your sides at the same shoulder height as shown in photo.

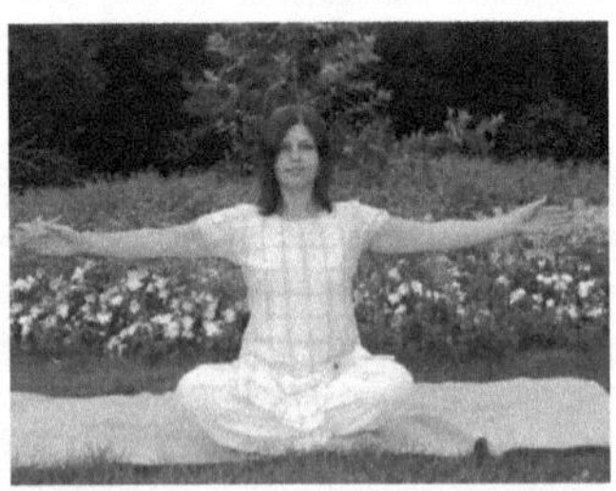

Step2: Now exhaling slowly and bring your arms together with palms touching each other.

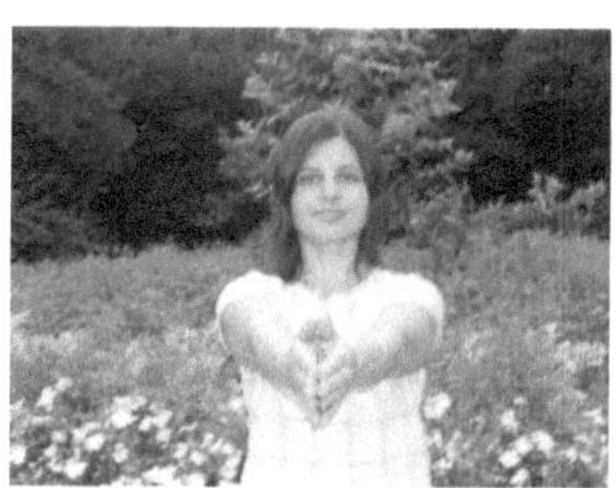

This is one round. Please practice 5 rounds and rest for few breaths after that.

Note: *Please remember arms should move slowly with full awareness of your breath & breath movement is synchronised with arms movement.*

This exercise can also be practised while sitting on chair.

Exercise 10
Hand Stretch movement

Preparation: Either stand straight with feet together or sit in a cross leg position, interlocking the fingers and placing the palms on the chest as shown in picture.

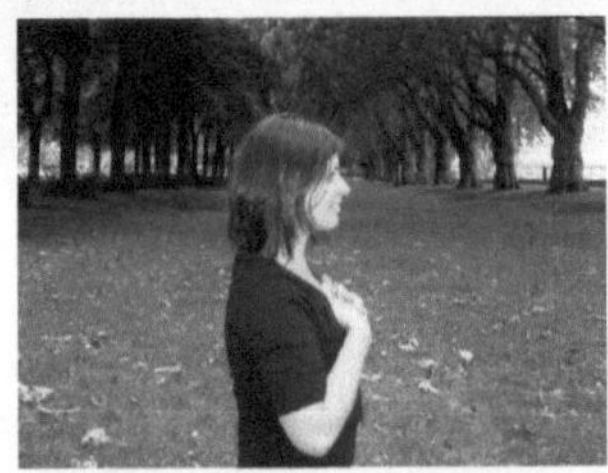

Step 1: Now inhale and stretch out the arms while palms facing outside as shown in the picture.

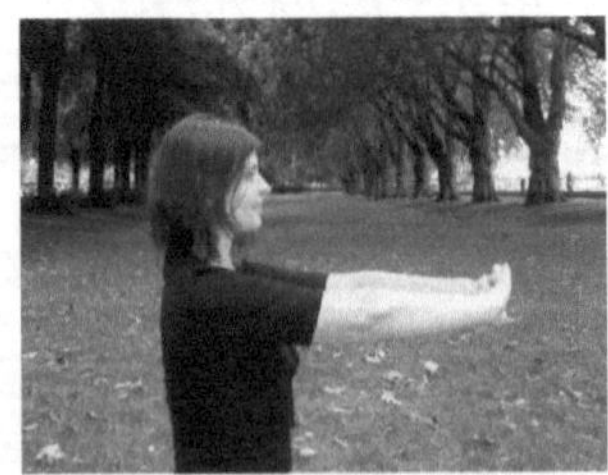

Step 2: Exhale and bring the palms back on chest.

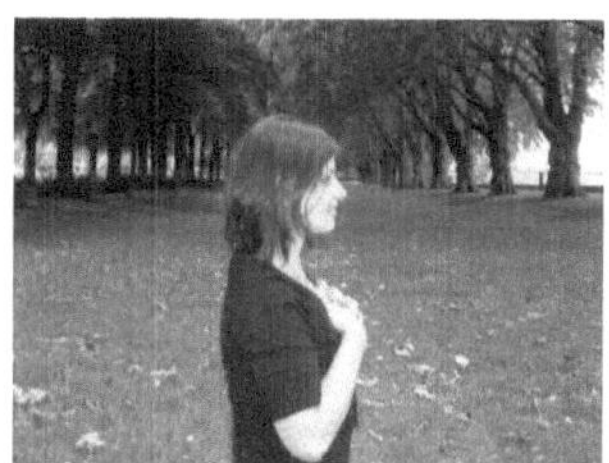

This is one round. Please practice about 5 to 10 rounds as per your comfort level. Never strain in any position.

Note: If tiredness is felt at any point during any gentle exercises, please lie down on your back on the floor for couple of minutes and practice deep breathing.

36

Exercise 11
Half butterfly posture

Preparation: Place yourself in a sitting position with your back straight (as much as possible) as shown in the picture below. Keep your left leg straight on floor and place the right foot on the floor beside the left knee.

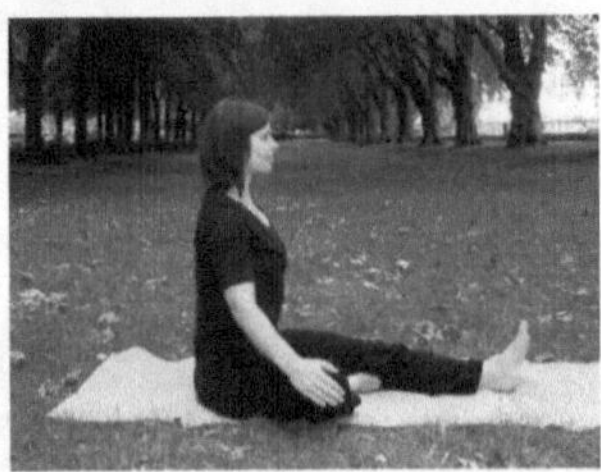

Your left palm on the floor provides you balance and right palm holds the right knee.

Step1: Now inhale and lift your right knee up with the help of your right palm.

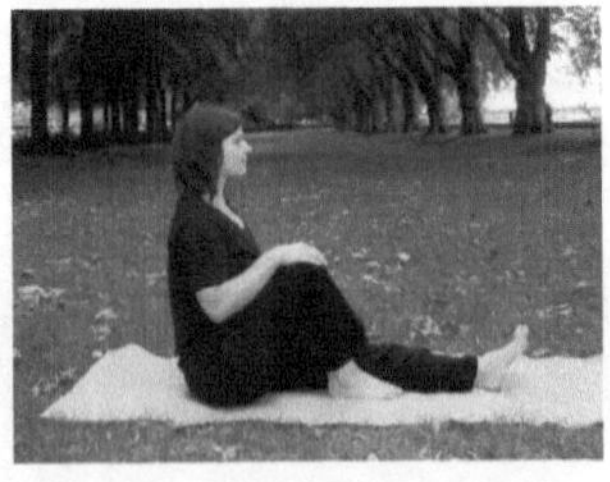

Step 2: As you exhale bring your right knee down with the help of your right palm.

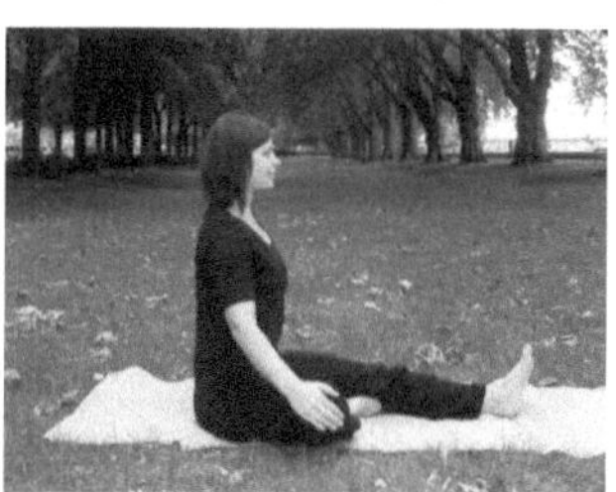

You can practice this between 5 to 10 times without straining yourself. Then repeat the same movement with the other leg.

Benefits:

This is excellent exercise for loosening knee and hip joints.

Note: *After practicing this half butterfly exercise please always do single knee bending exercise which is explained next.*

Exercise 12
Single Knee bending exercise

Preparation: Sit on the floor with legs straight and inhale deeply.

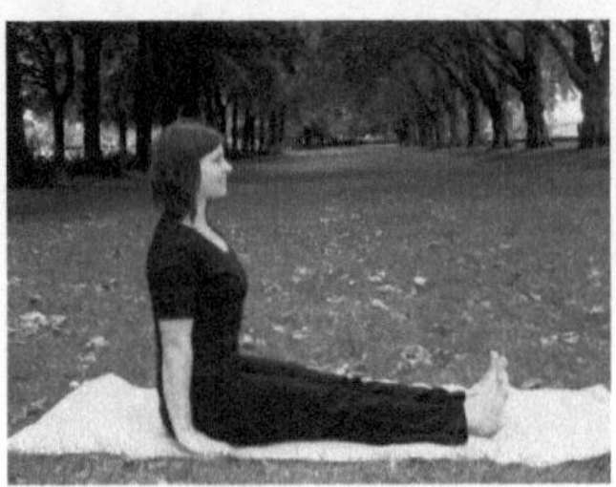

Step1: Now exhale while bending your right knee and keep you head and spine straight as shown in the picture.

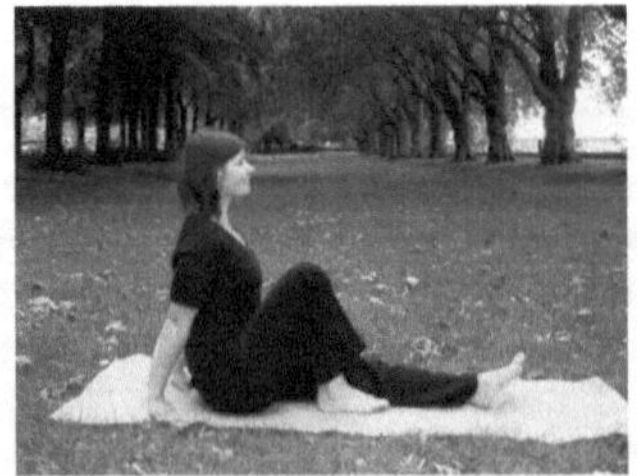

Step2: While inhaling straighten the right leg back to a straight position.

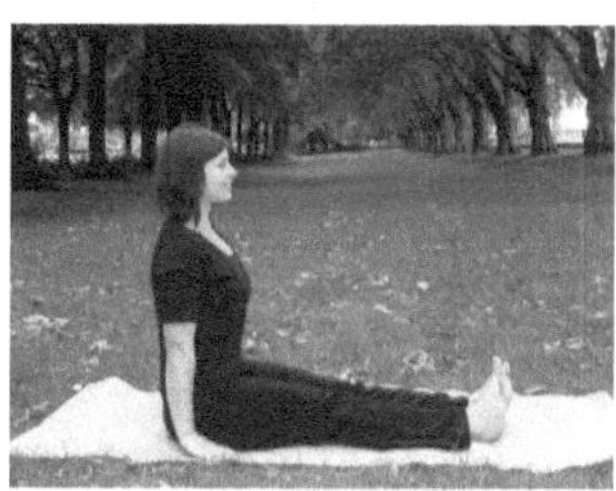

Now repeat it with left knee as well.

This is one round.

Practice 5 rounds.

Exercise 13
Ankle stretching exercise

Preparation: Sit on the floor with your legs straight and back straight.

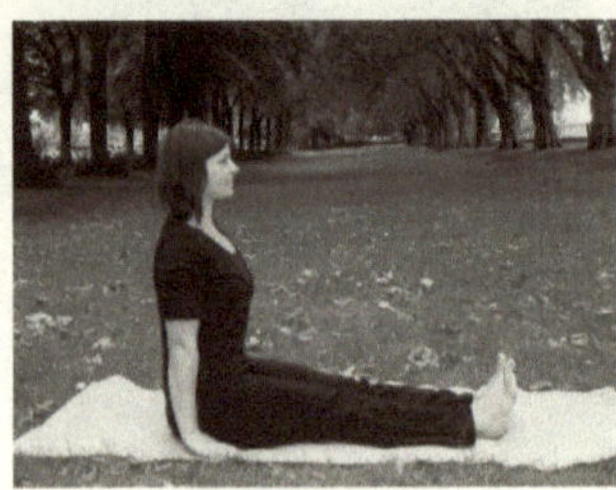

Step1. As you inhale move your both feet down as shown in the picture.

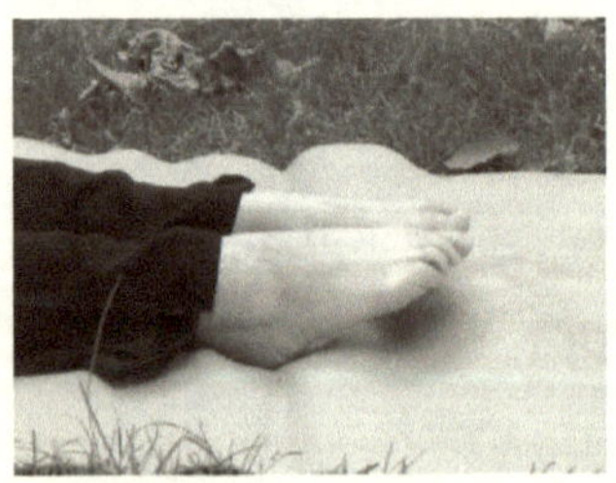

Step2. As you exhale move your both feet back, towards you, as shown in the picture.

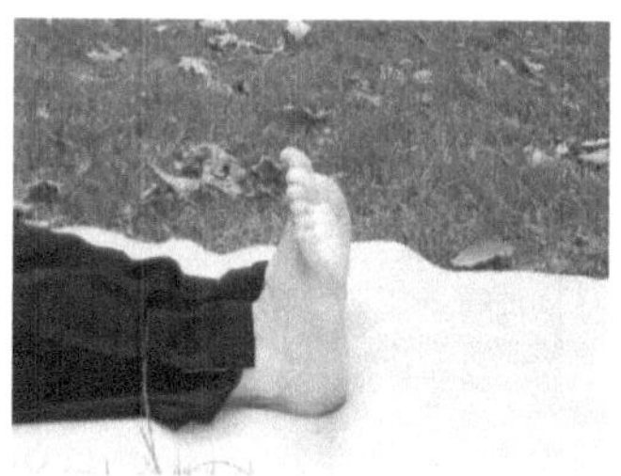

This completes one round.

Practice 5 rounds.

(If you find it difficult to sit on floor you can do this gentle movement while sitting on chair as well).

Exercise 14
Ankle rotation

Preparation: Sit on the floor with your legs straight and back straight.

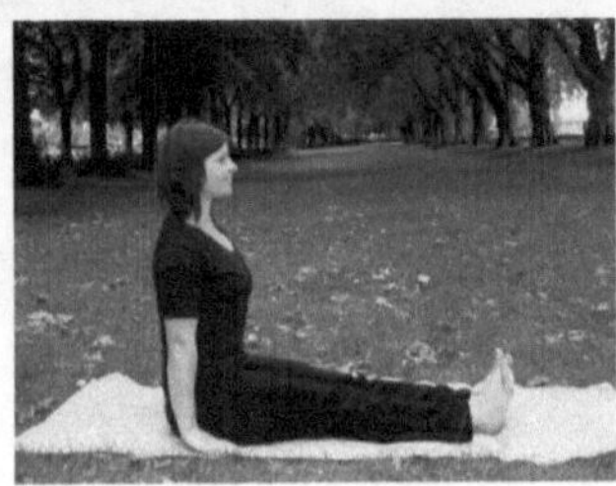

Rotate both feet in clockwise direction and be aware that you are not moving your knees.

Step1. As you exhale rotate your feet downward.

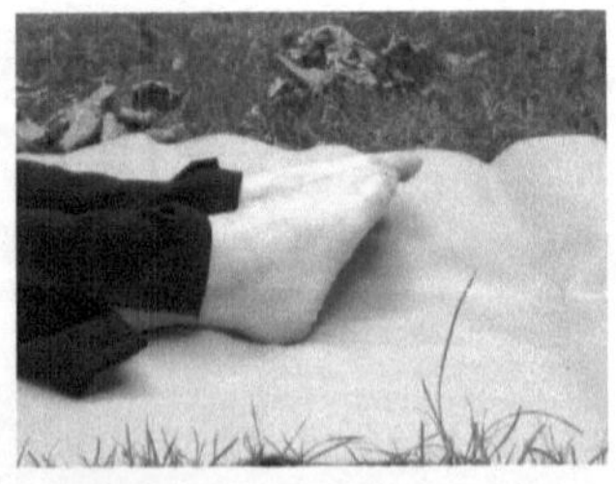

Step2. As you inhale rotate your feet upward.

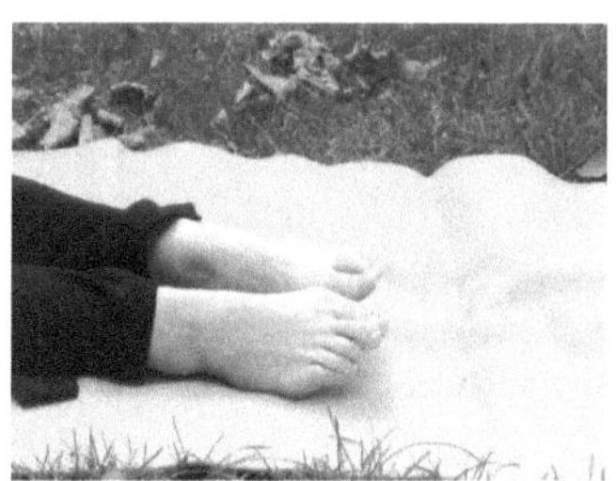

You can practice 5 to 10 times rotating both feet in clockwise direction and after that rotate both feet 5 to 10 times in anti clockwise direction.

Benefits:

This movement relieves tiredness and cramps from legs.

Exercise 15

Toe bending

Preparation: Sit on the floor with your legs straight and back straight.

Place your hands on the floor besides you and try to make your back as straight as possible as shown in the picture.

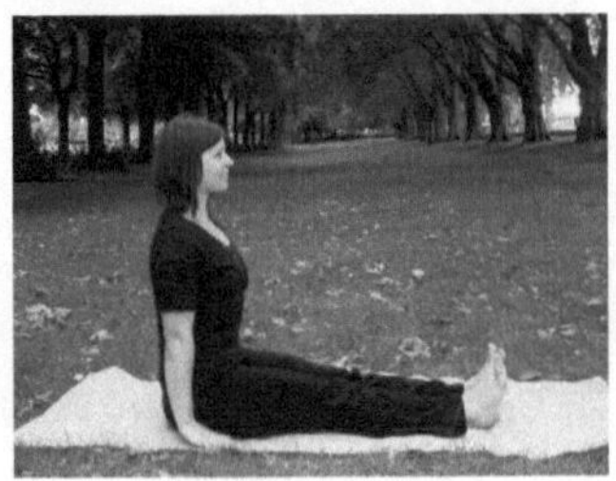

Step1. As you inhale bend your toes forward, away from you as shown in the picture.

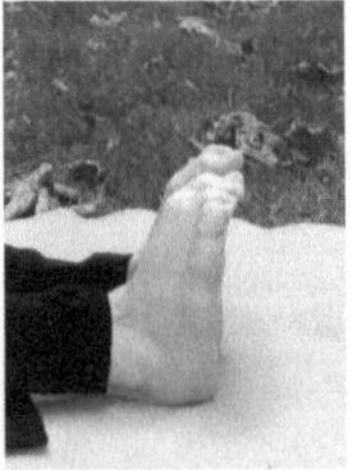

Step2. As you exhale bend your toes back, towards you as shown in the picture.

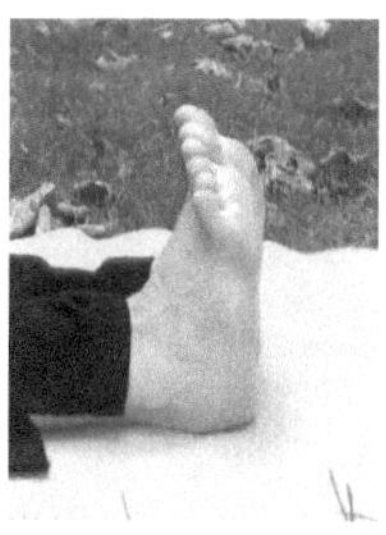

This completes one round.

Practice 10 to 20 rounds.

Exercise 16
Cat Stretch

Come up in a position as shown in the picture below with your knees under your hips and your palms under your shoulders.

Your wrists, elbows and shoulders are in line and perpendicular to the floor. Centre your head in a neutral position, eyes looking at the floor (picture below).

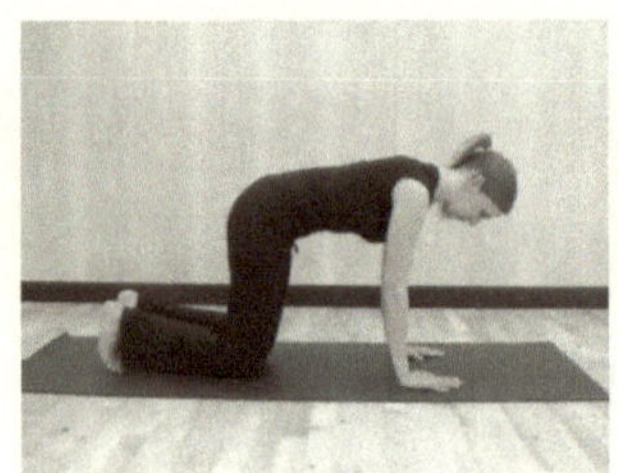

While inhaling slowly and deeply, lift your head up and bring your spine down within your comfort level as shown in the picture below.

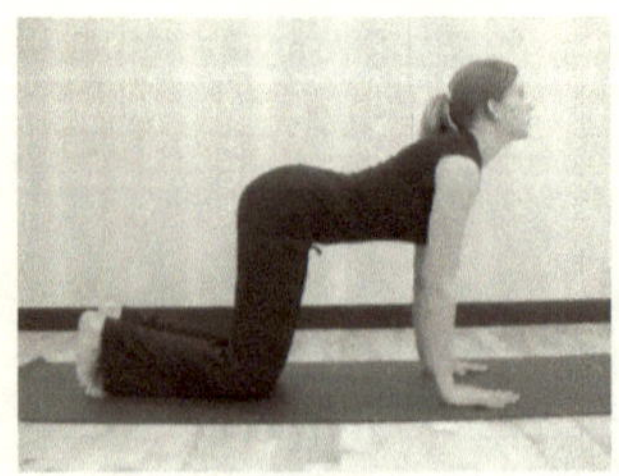

As you slowly exhale bring you head down and round your spine toward the ceiling and contract your abdomen as shown in the picture below.

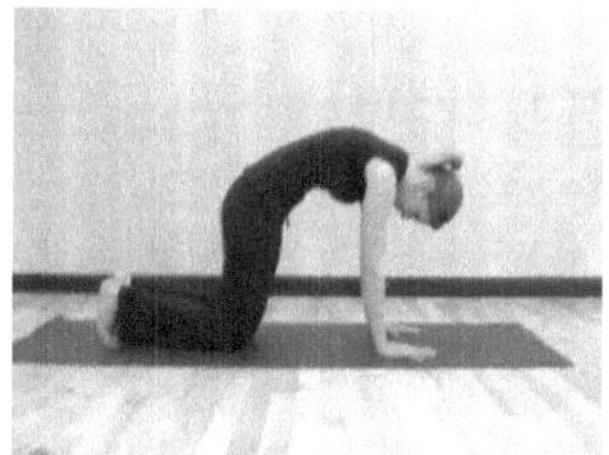

This inhalation and exhalation complete one round. You can practice 5 to 10 rounds.

This is a very good exercise for improving flexibility of the spine and it is especially helpful after long hours of sitting in the office or driving to release stiffness from the back.

Caution:

In case of neck injury and pregnancy, please practice it under guidance of an experienced yoga teacher only.

Exercise17
Spinal Twist

Step by step method:

Preparation: Lie flat on your back with your legs straight and palms facing down.

Step 1: Bend the right knee and place the right foot on the floor by the left knee.

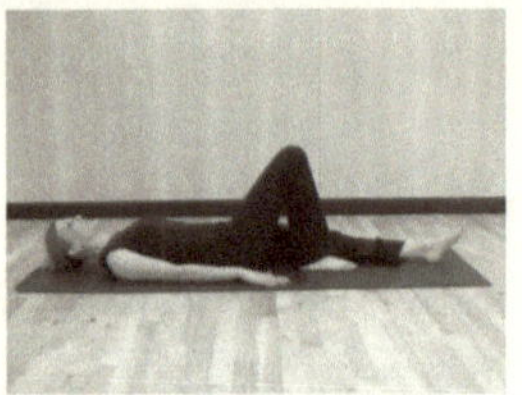

Then place your left hand on top of the right knee, as shown in picture.

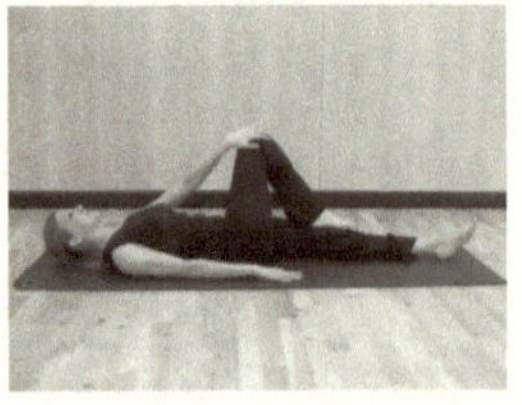

Step 2: As you exhale, bring your right knee down towards the floor on the left side of your body, turning around 45 degree left side or half way and turn your head to the right side of your body.

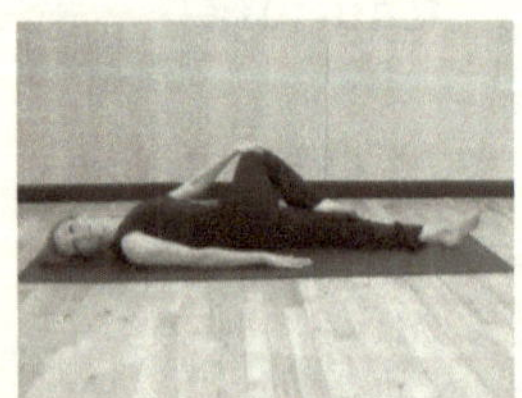

(Note: *In this position your right arm and your right shoulder should be touching the floor comfortably*).

Now hold this posture for about 30 seconds and keep breathing naturally.

Step 3: As you inhale slowly return to the centre.

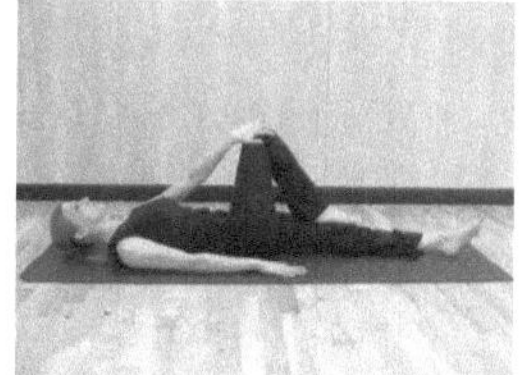

Step 4: Repeat on the other side (this completes one round).

Benefits: This yoga posture helps in releasing tightness and tiredness in the lower back and it is excellent for you, if you have a job which involves sitting on the chair for long hours.

Caution: If you experience pain at any stage, please make sure that you are not overstretching.

50

Exercise 18
Diaphragmatic Breathing

Deep abdominal breathing or diaphragmatic breathing happens because of action of diaphragm. In this breathing exercise during inhalation, the diaphragm moves downward, which pushes abdominal down and outward and during exhalation the diaphragm moves upward and abdomen moves inward. Abdominal breathing is the most natural and efficient breathing. *One can observe a little baby breath since the moment of his/her birth and it is diaphragmatic breathing only.*

<u>For performing or learning abdominal breathing</u>

First lie down flat on your back and relax your whole body. Check yourself if there is any tension in any of your body part and if you find any tightness just release it. Now take your awareness towards your breath.

Next observe your natural breath and make sure you are not controlling it but only observing it.

Now place your left hand on the abdomen on your navel area.

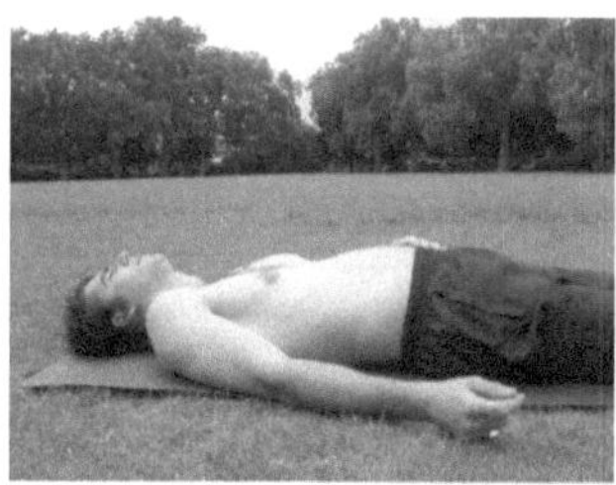

(Abdomen position during inhalation)

If you are breathing naturally through your abdomen, your left hand (which is above abdomen) would move up with inhalation and down with exhalation.

Try to take your breath down deeper and deeper into the lungs so that you feel the abdomen lifting as you breathe in and falling as you breathe out.

Gradually, you would notice that the abdomen is moving more firmly, and the chest moving less. As abdominal breathing becomes easier to you, try to let your breathing become *slower, deeper* and *smoother*.

The slow, deep and smooth breath would bring relaxation to the body and mind. This is the breathing pattern you can use at all times, while at rest or at work. Practice it until it becomes natural and unconscious.

Note: Practicing this deep breathing exercise everyday for minimum 5 minutes helps in relaxation and releasing stress.

I highly recommend everyday practice of this exercise.

Cautions:

Make sure that there are no jerks in flow of your breath. The flow of your breath should be smooth and without any noise.

Gentle Yoga practice record

I would like to recommend that for your good health please practice Gentle yoga everyday and after practice please mark your progress in the record below.

Starting date ....

Week 1	Sun	Mon	Tue	Wed	Thu	Fri	Sat
Gentle Yoga Practice							
Week 2	Sun	Mon	Tue	Wed	Thu	Fri	Sat
Gentle Yoga Practice							
Week 3	Sun	Mon	Tue	Wed	Thu	Fri	Sat
Gentle Yoga Practice							
Week 4	Sun	Mon	Tue	Wed	Thu	Fri	Sat
Gentle Yoga Practice							

After week 4 what improvement do you feel, please write in the box below

Our Published book:

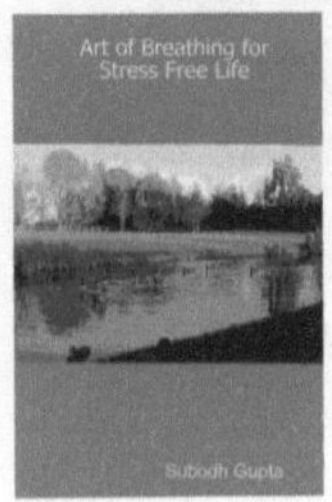

Art of Breathing *for* Stress free Life

The Only book on human breathing techniques for managing stress with clearly illustrated photographs and practical instructions. This book is ideal for busy people who lead a hectic life style.

Paperback/£4.95/ 56 pages

7 Food Habits for Weight Loss *Forever*

Stay Healthy and Slim *Forever*

"For anybody who wants to lose weight and gain health forever"

"*Managing perfect body weight is not a complicated rocket science. Our body is made up of food which we eat during our day to day life. If we are overweight or obese at the moment then one thing is certain that the food which we eat is not good.*"

Healthy Food Habits = Good Health + Perfect Body Weight *Forever*

ISBN 978-0-9556882-0-1
Page 68 / Soft Cover / £4.95

India Culture and Travel scams

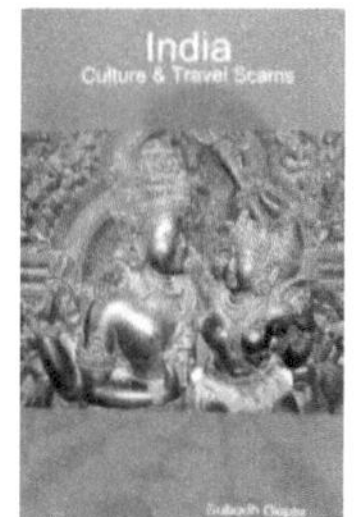

"The only book on travel scams targeted at western tourists in India"

This is a practical book about understanding Indian culture and travel scams in India and is based on real life experiences.

This book will help you to avoid embarrassing mistakes and prepare you to feel confident in unfamiliar situations. Content in this book includes Indian social customs, their perception about Western women, their religion, what motivates them, travel scams targeted at Western tourists and of course what not to discuss with Indians, etc.

Page 112/Paper Back / £5.95
ISBN 978-0-9556882-6-3

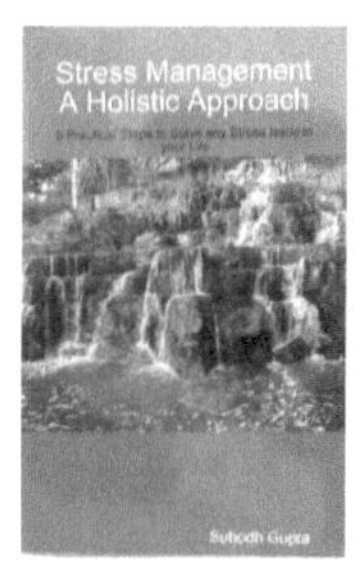

Stress Management A Holistic Approach
5 steps plan to manage Stress in your life

Many illnesses such as diabetes, migraine, asthma, ulcer and even cancer arise because of excessive Stress over the period of time.

You may have any kind of problem or issue in your life, once you follow the 5 steps described in this book you are on your way to Stress free life. If there is a problem then there has to be a solution and this book is all about solution.

ISBN 978-0-9556882-1-8
Page 80 / Soft Cover / £4.95

All our books are also available at Amazon.com, Barnes and Nobles